Table of Contents

Introduction

It's relatively easy to go plant-based or vegan, especially if it's short term. For example, veganuary encourages people to go vegan for the month of January and over 250,000 people tried it in 2019. But doing it well and making long term changes, well, that's a different story. Type in 'vegan' on YouTube and you will come across some people saying whilst vegan they ran into issues. It's said that any changes to a person's diet, for a short while you will feel amazing but over time, if not done properly the cracks can start to appear.

I've been plant-based for 8 years and I have thrived. Moreover I've helped hundreds do the same. One of the key questions I get asked is how I got muscular, lean and strong whilst being plant based for so long. I always give the same answer…

In this book I am going to take you through one of the most important concepts for health, nutrients. Nutrients are substances that provide nourishment essential for the maintenance of life and for growth. In the later chapters I'm going to go through each nutrient the body requires and where you can get said nutrient on a plant-based vegan diet.

Before we get into that, it's always good to give some background information.

Plant-based or vegan diet

The terms plant-based and vegan are used interchangeably but there is a slight difference between them. Being plant-based does not necessarily mean you are vegan and vice versa. Donald Watson coined the term 'vegan' in 1944 when he co-founded the Vegan Society in the UK. Since then, veganism has grown expeditiously to be a worldwide phenomenon.

The short definition of a vegan is someone who does not eat or use animal products. On the other hand, a person who is plant-based eats a diet consisting mostly or entirely of foods derived from plants. So although there are crossovers, simply put, vegan is a lifestyle and plant-based is a diet.

Some vegans do not care about the health or quality of the foods they consume as long as it does not harm animals whereas plant-based individuals focus on plant derived whole-foods. Additionally, vegans do not wear leather or eat honey but some plant-based individuals may do so. So although you can be both, it's good to get an understanding of both terms before we dive deeper into this book.

I personally try not to use labels anymore but if I was describing how I eat I'll use the term plant-based whereas if a stranger was to describe how I eat, they will probably say vegan. So does it really matter? In all honesty, I am Dungutarian (this term will catch on one day).

No matter what term you use to describe yourself the important thing is ensuring you get the nutrients the body requires. From vegetarian to carnivore, the body cares more about the quality of the nutrients you consume rather than the labels you put on yourself. This book will ensure you understand what nutrients the body requires and potential sources of these nutrients that you can add to your diet.

Going plant-based, the truth

Towards the end of 2011 I found the curiosity I once had as a child. All children go through a 'why stage' at around 3 years old. During the why stage, asking why is a sign of curiosity and wanting to understand the world around them. As we grow up, life seems to reduce our curiosity, until some of us just accept things for what they are without questioning why.

I'm not exactly sure what sparked me finding my curiosity again, was it the fact that I was battling with keloids on my ear. Or because I was doing a lot of self experimenting. One experiment was I cut out foods I ate everyday for a month and I was mindful of how my body responded. For example, I used to eat full fat milk, cornflakes and bread everyday, without fail. YES, EVERYDAY.

During the experiment I cut these foods out for one month. In that month I noticed my pimples cleared and my face was noticeably smoother and glowing. I remember asking myself is there a link between milk and spots?

Also during these same times I was trying to heal my keloid. For those who don't know what a keloid is, a keloid is an area of irregular fibrous tissue formed at the site of a scar or injury. This tissue can keep growing and in my case, my ear looked like it had a huge earring dangling off it. This growth is called a keloid. I remember learning how wheat and peanut butter can inflame a keloid and lead to more growth.

These experiences further sparked my interest in understanding how food affected the body. Couple that with unlimited access to Google and an intense desire to understand the body, nutrition, food and disease. I made a slow decision to start cutting out foods starting with red meat. At the time I didn't know any of the terms vegan or plant-based, I just wanted to eat what I thought was as natural as possible.

Now, I've been eating a full plant based diet for over 8 years now. Initially, one thing that I found key to optimising my health and physique in my new diet was ensuring I knew what vitamins, minerals, fats and proteins were essential to me.

In the beginning I researched the body, what it needs, food sources and crafted a personal diet that I thought works well for me; not much variety but foods that give me all the nutrients I need. A friend asked me for some information on these food sources and back in 2012/ 2013 I always went overboard with answers to questions I got asked (I had a 'Ask Dungu' series on twitter at the time where I answered health questions). On this occasion I put the information on foods into an excel sheet, spending time carefully curating information from some of the best sources.

Over time this document grew into an easy to read excel sheet that covers each nutrient, mineral, vitamin, protein and fat, their benefits, deficiency symptoms and more. That document has now grown into this guide. Crazy how things work out right. The first version of this book made its way to over 10,000 people and I hope this new book reaches more. And with your help, I'm sure it will. Don't forget to leave a review on Amazon, it really helps the cause.

Understanding nutrients

What is the purpose of food? Most of us would reply to that question with keywords like energy, nourish and fuel. But how does this process work and if we eat something that does not nourish the body or provide energy is that still food? If you feel tired after eating, can it be said that the food did not nourish the body effectively?

The reason for this line of questioning is to help spark some curiosity and connections. These are the questions I asked myself in 2011 that allowed me to see food as more than just something that tastes good or makes me feel happy but to actually see it as fuel. And that fuel is nutrients.

Nutrients are molecules in food that all organisms need to make energy, grow, develop, repair and reproduce. When we consume food, the food is digested and the nutrients are broken down into basic parts to be used by the body. The two main types of nutrients are macronutrients and micronutrients.

Macronutrients are broken down into three main categories, these include carbohydrates, protein and fat. Whereas micronutrients are broken down into two categories; vitamins and minerals.

Most people are aware of the macronutrients the body needs such as fats, carbohydrates and proteins. But as long as a person eats, it's hard to be deficient in macronutrients, on the other hand micronutrients are crucial to the wellbeing of the body and even one deficiency can lead to a roller coaster of problems.

For example, have you ever had a great night's sleep and woke up still tired? Or had a headache randomly? Experienced pins and needles? Chances are that these are symptoms of a micronutrient deficiency.

Making changes, the right way

To avoid deficiencies and issues whilst adopting a plant-based diet, we are going to discuss the two ways to go about making changes and their pros and cons.

The first way to adopt a plant-based vegan diet is the light switch method; you drop everything and make the switch instantly. The second is the step by step method. Choosing which works for you depends on what kind of person you are and what you are trying to achieve, for example your why.

Your why could be you want to make a lifestyle change and reduce meat consumption to better yourself or you want to try meatless for a new years resolution.

The first option is the light switch method. This is a complete overhaul of your diet. This is useful for some, especially if you're only going vegan for a certain period of time or that's what works best for you. You're the kind of person to always give something your all and when you make your mind up about something, you run with it. If that's the case, still try to learn more about your new diet, this builds confidence that you made the right decision.

If you want to make a switch for life, this switch requires knowledge and lots of it. Knowledge builds motivation to make the changes. Knowledge helps you understand why you're doing it. The why keeps you going through tough times and it takes roughly 6 weeks to form a habit and make it a lifestyle. The knowledge will change how you see food thus leading to long term changes.

The biggest mistake most people make is that they make changes without replacing the foods with other more wholesome food. This can be a shock to the body. I've seen people go the absolute extremes. For example, when they first go vegan they cut out all the meat and then start eating raw vegetables. You may feel you're doing the body good, but this shock may lead to very frequent visits to the toilet or even stomach cramps.

Furthermore, without understanding what foods to replace with what, a person may reduce their protein consumption and thus lose muscle mass during their initial cut. Especially if they do not have a good understanding of calories, something we will discuss later.

The second way to adopt a plant-based diet is a steady cut (step by step). With a steady cut, you cut out red meats and continue to eat white flesh meats and fish. Then you minimise white flesh, for example, you eat chicken once a week and continue with fish. After a while you make a decision to cut it all out. This may take you 3 weeks or 6 months, there is no time limit as long as you're progressing.

At each stage you're adding wholesome nutrient dense foods to your diet, you're creating new recipes with the foods listed in this book and you're reevaluating how you feel at each stage. This is where a food journal or diary comes in. If you get a good understanding of how you feel, you can have the confidence to move to the next stage. For example, do you have more energy, are you sleeping better or even lighter, these are some of the feelings that allow you to progress.

Whichever method works best for you, go for it. But remember, do not blindly follow people and their beliefs, keep the curiosity of a child. Periodically, question your beliefs, ask yourself if you made the right decision, take in new information and make decisions based on having all the facts. That's how you grew before and that's how you will continuously grow. Having a lifestyle choice as part of your identity is good to spread a message but this can also cloud your judgement and reduce your curiosity. Something to think about.

"Stay hungry, stay young, stay foolish, stay curious, and above all, stay humble because just when you think you got all the answers, is the moment when some bitter twist of fate in the universe will remind you that you very much don't." - **Tom Hiddleston**

Calories

Although this book is about nutrients, understanding calories is important for anyone trying a new diet. In this chapter we're going to talk about calories, calorie breakdown and how to work out how much calories you need. Also, we'll briefly cover how to gain and lose weight using this information.

What are calories?

A calorie is a unit of energy. Essentially, it describes how much energy your body could get from a particular food or drink.. To understand how many calories the body needs and how many calories a food is providing you, it's best to look at some food labels.

Nutrition Facts

Serving Size 1 cup (228g)
Servings Per Container 2

Amount Per Serving

Calories 250   Calories from Fat 110

% Daily Value*

Total Fat 12g	18%
Saturated Fat 3g	15%
Trans Fat 3g	
Cholesterol 30mg	10%
Sodium 470mg	20%
Total Carbohydrate 31g	10%
Dietary Fiber 0g	0%
Sugars 5g	
Protein 5g	

Vitamin A	4%
Vitamin C	2%
Calcium	20%
Iron	4%

* Percent Daily Values are based on a 2,000 calorie diet. Your Daily Values may be higher or lower depending on your calorie needs.

	Calories	2,000	2,500
Total Fat	Less than	65g	80g
Sat Fat	Less than	20g	25g
Cholesterol	Less than	300mg	300mg
Sodium	Less than	2,400mg	2,400mg
Total Carbohydrate		300g	375g
Dietary Fiber		25g	30g

A food label will show the amount of energy (calories) in the food, this either tends to be shown as per 100 grams or per serving. Sometimes energy is presented in three ways on average, KJ which stands for Kilojoules, Kcal short for kilocalories or cal, short for calories. Calories and kilocalories tend to be used interchangeably.

Kilojoules are the metric measurement of calories and another measurement of energy. Depending on where you are in the world, you'll either use one or the other but it's more than likely you see calories on your food labels.

The calories on the label is made up of all the macronutrients beneath it. Essentially the calories are made up of fat, protein and carbohydrates. So a 100 calorie food might be made up of 30 calories from fat, 50 calories from carbohydrates and 20 calories from protein. It's worth noting that micronutrients are needed only in very small amounts and tend not provide any calories.

On the food label where you see - of which saturates, this means out of the fats in the food, this is how many grams of it are saturated. If you minus the saturates from the total fat you will see how much unsaturated fat is in the food. Similarly with carbohydrates, if you minus how much sugars are there from the total -

carbohydrates, you will see how much complex carbs and fibres are in the food (sometimes fibres are shown in its own column).

To understand what calorie goal is right for you in your new diet, you need to understand how to calculate how much calories your body requires.

Calculating calories

Start with the Basal metabolic rate (BSR). BSR is the amount of energy per unit time that a person needs to keep the body processes functioning at rest. These processes include breathing, blood circulation, controlling body temperature, cell growth, brain and nerve function, and contraction of muscles.

To calculate this you will need this formula:

Men
Basal Metabolic Rate (BMR) = 66 + (13.8 x weight in kg) + (5 x height in cm) - (6.8 x age in years)

Women: Basal Metabolic Rate (BMR) = 655 + (9.6 x weight in kg) + (1.8 x height in cm) - (4.7 x age in years)

BMR x 1.3 = weight maintenance calories

Another way to calculate maintenance calories is by multiplying your weight in KG by 30 calories.

Calorie deficit and surplus

On a plant-based diet the calorie density within food can change, you tend to have less calorie dense foods but more nutrient dense foods. In this chapter you will see how to put on or lose weight with some quick maths.

But first, what is a calorie deficit? A calorie deficit is consuming less calories than your body requires to maintain the same body weight. On the other hand a calorie surplus is the opposite, it's a state in which you eat more calories than you burn.

So let's say your maintenance calorie (calculated in previous chapter) is 3000 calories and you eat 3300 calories a day, you're in a surplus and you will gain weight. If you eat 2700 per day, you're in a calorie deficit and you will lose weight.

The question is how much of a surplus or deficit should you be in. To understand how much, it's useful to know that 1kg of weight is around 7000 calories. So if you want to put 1kg of weight on in 2 weeks that's 7000 / 14 days. You'll need to consume an extra 500 calories a day.

To lose 2kg you need to be doing the opposite and consume 500 calories less a day. The average calorie surplus or deficit recommended is between 200 to 450 depending.

With a good understanding of nutrients and calories, you can conquer the world, attain any physique you want and optimise your health. Next you will understand that not all calories are equal, calorie dense foods and nutrient density is the key to achieving success on a plant-based diet.

Calorie dense

Calorie dense foods are foods that have a high amount of calories per weight of food.

Low calorie dense foods tend to have less fat (fat is 9 calories per gram) and more fiber. They will make you feel full but it will be harder to hit your calorie goal as high-fiber foods provide volume but low calories, meaning you will feel full with fewer calories. Also, the body cannot digest fiber, it just passes through you and aids digestion.

Think of your stomach like a muscle. Low calorie dense foods fill up the stomach quickly but these foods do not have as many calories in them. Whereas high calorie dense foods take up less space but have higher calories.

When the stomach is filled with large meals three times a day, the amount your stomach walls can stretch increases - allowing you to start eating more per meal. In other words, the more you eat, the more you can eat and thus get the calories your body needs to gain weight.

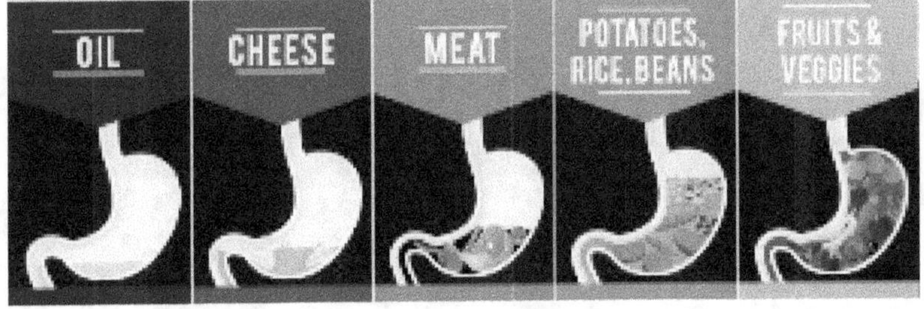

My top foods for weight gain are nuts, legumes, avocados, good fats, plantain, sweet potatoes and chickpeas. Understanding the calorie density concept should give you an understanding of why people lose weight when adopting a new plant-based diet. This is because the majority of vegetables are low calorie dense, so people eat them and fill full but are in a calorie deficit and thus not able to build muscle or gain weight.

The key thing is to ensure that although the food is calorie dense, it's also nutrient dense, as nutrients are what will actually nourish the body.

Nutrients dense

Nutrient density identifies the amount of beneficial nutrients such as vitamins, fats, minerals, lean proteins within a food in proportion to its calorie content, weight or amount of detrimental nutrients.

Within the subgroups of vitamins and minerals there are water soluble vitamins and fat soluble vitamins. Water soluble vitamins are vitamins that dissolve in water, these include vitamins B6, C and folic acid. Fat soluble vitamins are vitamins that can dissolve in fats and oils, these include Vitamin A, D, E and K. Some key essential minerals include calcium, magnesium and potassium. Picking foods that are both calorie and nutrient dense allows you gain the most of a plant-based diet.

As you read over the nutrition guide you will find similar foods in different categories. It's worth noting that the foods listed in this book are not an exhaustive list, they are foods that I tend to eat personally as I've found them to be both nutrient and calorie dense. Especially for bodybuilding. Ensure you keep experimenting, learn new foods, try new recipes and if there are any foods you want me to add to the next versions of this book, just email them to me via paul@dungubook.com.

Something that may help you is to keep a food journal. For 3 days and write down how to eat but also note how you feel after eating. Note how you feel immediately and after an hour or two. Are energetic, sleepy, hungry again or bloated? This is because different people have different intolerances for certain foods and some people are sensitive to what some nutritionists call 'antinutrients'.

Antinutrients

Antinutrients can block the absorption of nutrients. Antinutrients can be found in many plant-based foods. It's thought that these compounds are in these nuts, seeds and plants to ward them from bacterial infections and being eaten by insects.

Antinutrients is where some people go wrong whilst trying out a plant-based diet. They end up feeling bloated or getting stomach upset and not understanding why.

The common antinutrients are gluten, glucosinolates, lectins, oxalates, phytates, saponins, and tannins.

- **Glucosinolates** can prevent the absorption of iodine, which may then interfere with thyroid function and cause goiter.

- **Lectins** in legumes can interfere with the absorption of calcium, iron, phosphorus, and zinc.
- **Oxalates** in green leafy vegetables and tea can bind to calcium and reduce absorption.
- **Phytates** in whole grains, seeds, legumes, some nuts—can decrease the absorption of iron, zinc, magnesium, and calcium.
- **Tannins** in tea, legumes, wines and coffee can decrease iron absorption.

So what's the deal, should you avoid them or are there ways to reduce antinutrients? There is still a lot of research in this field and a lot of conflicting information.

Some parts of the antinutrient research are slightly agreed on like many antinutrients like phytates, lectins, and glucosinolates can be removed or deactivated by soaking, sprouting, or boiling the food before eating. Some say eating a wide variety of foods and smaller portions helps combat potential issues. For example, instead of two cups of lentils or a large lentil portion, eat one normal portion with some plantain.

Studies on vegetarians who eat diets high in plant foods containing antinutrients do not generally show deficiencies in iron and zinc, so the body may be adapted to the presence of antinutrients. Also I believe some of us are intolerant to some antinutrients, for example, some people are intolerant to gluten.

It may be worth doing an intolerance test and eating a wide variety of foods to see how you react to them. I added this chapter in so you can be aware of it and spark some curiosity for further research.

Remember there are plenty of options, there are over 20,000 species of edible plants in the world yet fewer than 20 species provide 90% of our food. There are hundreds of less well known edible plants from all around the world which are both delicious and nutritious. So, be an explorer, a food explorer.

Without further adieu, let's get into the nutrient guide.

Vitamins

[**vahy**-t*uh*-min; *British also* **vit**-*uh*-min]

Vitamins are all needed by the body and are necessary for energy production, immune function, blood clotting and other functions.

Choline

RDI: 550 mg

DEFINITION

Choline is a micronutrient that is important for good liver function, brain development, nerve function, muscle movement, energy levels and maintaining a healthy metabolism.

FOODS I'D RECOMMEND

- Pistachios nuts (1 cup - 87.82 mg)
- Navy Beans (1 cup - 81.35 mg)
- Chickpeas (1 Cup - 70.19 mg)
- Split Peas (1 Cup - 64 mg)
- Teff (1 cup - 25.3 mg)
- Collard greens (1 cup - 61 mg)
- Cauliflower (1 serving - 24 mg)

- Mushrooms (½ cup - 58 mg)
- Quinoa (1 cup - 43 mg)

BENEFITS

- Used to create acetylcholine which is important for brain health
- Heart health
- Boost mood

DEFICIENCY SYMPTOMS

- Low energy levels of fatigue
- Memory loss
- Cognitive decline
- Learning disabilities
- Muscle aches
- Nerve damage
- Mood changes or disorders.

RELATES TO

B complex Vitamins and Folate

Lutein and Zeaxanthin

RDI: 6mg and 2mg

DEFINITION

Lutein and zeaxanthin are structurally very similar.
Lutein is important to eye health.

FOODS I'D RECOMMEND

- Broccoli (1 cup - 2.7 mg)
- Kale (1 cup - 20 mg)
- Spinach (1 cup - 8 mg)

BENEFITS

- Filter harmful high-energy blue wavelengths
- Help protect and maintain healthy eyes
- Powerful antioxidants

- Anti ageing

- Anti-inflammatory

DEFICIENCY SYMPTOMS

Deficiency of lutein and zeaxanthin can increase risk of:

- The risk of inflammatory polyarthritisIncreased risk of breast cancer

- Increased risk of prostate cancer

- Increased risk of colon cancer

- Increased risk of cervical cancer

- Human papilloma virus persistence

- Type 2 diabetes

- Liver issues

- Alzheimer's disease

Lycopene

RDI: Between 8-21 mg

DEFINITION

Lycopene gives fruits and vegetables a red or pink colour.

FOODS I'D RECOMMEND

Most pink and red fruits contain lycopene. Some of these fruits include

- Sun-Dried tomatoes - (100 g - 45.9 mg)
- Watermelon (100 g - 4.5 mg)
- Grapefruit - (100 g - 1.1 mg)
- Guavas (100 g - 5.2 mg)
- Papaya (100 g - 1.8 mg)

BENEFITS

- Powerful antioxidant

- Beneficial for muscle repair

- May play a role in preventing cancer

- May play a role in preventing heart disease

- Aids heart health

- Help eyesight

- Good for brain health

- Contribute to stronger bones.

DEFICIENCY SYMPTOMS

There are no known symptoms of a lycopene deficiency.

Vitamin A

RDI: 0.7 mg for men, 0.6 mg for women

DEFINITION

Vitamin A, also known as retinol., is an important nutrient involved in the immune system, eye health, reproduction, and cellular communication. There are two different types of vitamin A. The first type, preformed vitamin A, is found in animal products. On the other hand, the second type, provitamin A, is found in plant-based products.

FOODS I'D RECOMMEND

- Spinach (1 cup - 1.14 mg)
- Carrots (½ cupt - 0.459 mg)
- Sweet Potatoes (1 whole - 1.4 mg)
- Red Peppers (1 cup - 0.114 mg)
- Mango (1 whole - 0.112 mg)

- Papaya (1 cup - 1.3 mg)
- Apricots (1 cup - 0.063 mg)

BENEFITS

- Protects the eyes
- Reduces certain cancer risks
- Supports bone health
- Boosts immune system
- Helps protect you from night blindness
- Beneficial for skin health

DEFICIENCY SYMPTOMS

- Dry Skin
- Dry eyes
- Night blindness
- Slow wound healing
- Dry lips and tongue

RELATES TO

Calcium and vitamin D are also essential for building strong, dense bones. Additionally, you can contribute to your vitamin A intake by including good sources of beta carotene in your diet, as this can be converted into vitamin A by the body.

It's worth noting that too much Vitamin A can be risky.

Vitamin B1 - Thiamin

RDI: 1.2 mg

DEFINITION

Vitamin B1, Thiamin, or sometimes spelt Thiamine, is an essential nutrient required by the body for maintaining cellular function. As with all B vitamins, it's a water soluble vitamin, it dissolves in water and is carried through the bloodstream. Whatever the body does not use is eliminated in urine and thus it needs to be acquired through food often.

FOODS I'D RECOMMEND

- Kelp seaweed (100 g - 0.05 mg)
- Lentils (1 cup - 0.34 mg *boiled)
- Chia seeds (100 g - 0.62 mg)
- Flax seeds (100 g - 1.64 mg)
- Teff (1 cup - 0.8 mg)

- Hemp seeds (100 g - 1.275 mg)

- Quinoa (100 g - 0.38 mg)

- Pistachio (100 g - 0.87 mg)

- Cashews (100 g - 0.42 mg)

- Cauliflower (1 cup - 0.05mg)

- Black beans (100 g - 0.192 mg)

BENEFITS

- Anti aging

- Muscle repair

- Energy

- Digestion

- Memory

- Red blood cells restoration

DEFICIENCY SYMPTOMS

- Severe fatigue
- Loss of appetite
- Irritability
- Muscular
- Pins and needle

Vitamin B2 - Riboflavin

RDI: 1.3 mg for men and 1.1 mg for women

DEFINITION

Vitamin B2, also known as Riboflavin, is an important nutrient that plays a role in helping your body produce (or unlock) energy and metabolism. Research suggests that a riboflavin deficiency may impair iron metabolism.

Vitamin B2 is also involved in utilising the energy from the nutrients we consume.

FOODS I'D RECOMMEND

- Almonds (100 g - 1.1 mg)
- Cashews (100 g - 0.06 mg)
- Mushrooms - (100 g - 0.5 mg)

- Spinach (100 g - 0.2 mg)
- Broccoli (100 g - 0.12 mg)
- Teff (1 cup - 0.5 mg)
- Quinoa (100 g - 0.39 mg)
- Avocados - (100 g - 0.1 mg)

BENEFITS

- Faster wound healing
- Anti-inflammatory
- May reduce migraines
- Good metabolism
- Energy

DEFICIENCY SYMPTOMS

- Fatigue
- Slowed growth
- Digestive problems
- Sores around the corners of the mouth
- Eye fatigue

- Swelling and soreness of the throat

- Sensitivity migraines

RELATES TO

Folate, Iron, Vitamin B6.

Vitamin B3 - Niacin

RDI: 16 mg for men and 14 mg for women

DEFINITION

Vitamin B3, or Niacin is used to describe also nicotinic acid, nicotinamide and niacinamide, these terms can be used interchangeably and mean one thing, vitamin B3. Niacin is an essential vitamin required for processing fat, DNA synthesis, cholesterol levels and it plays a role in regulation of glucose (blood sugar).

FOODS I'D RECOMMEND

- Brown rice (1 cup - 5.2 mg)
- Peanuts (100 g - 13.53 mg)
- Mushrooms (1 cup - 2.5 mg)
- Avocado (1 whole - 3.5 mg)
- Teff (1 cup - 6.5 mg)

- Chia seeds (1 oz - 2.5 mg)

- Almonds (100 g - 3.385 mg)

- Lentils (100 g - 2.605 mg)

BENEFITS

- Lowers LDL Cholesterol

- Boost brain function

- Beneficial for skin

- Anti-inflammatory

- Boosts Brain Function

- skin benefits

- Anti inflammatory

DEFICIENCY SYMPTOMS

- Irritability

- Poor concentration

- Headaches

- Memory loss

- Skin issues

- Anxiety
- Fatigue
- Lack of enthusiasm
- Depression
- Diarrhea

RELATES TO

Tryptophan helps increase niacin intake.

Vitamin B5 - Pantothenic Acid

RDI: 5 mg

DEFINITION

Vitamin B5 also known as Pantothenic Acid is critical to the manufacture of red blood cells, as well as sex and stress-related hormones produced in the adrenal glands.

FOODS I'D RECOMMEND

- Cauliflower
- Kale
- Broccoli
- Tomatoes
- Avocado
- Legumes
- Lentils

BENEFITS

- Create red blood cells
- Create hormones
- Healthy digestive tract
- Synthesise cholesterol
- Moisturising effects on the skin
- Reduces inflammation

DEFICIENCY SYMPTOMS

Rare but may include symptoms such as:

- Fatigue
- Insomnia
- Irritability
- Vomiting
- Stomach pains

RELATED TO

Process other vitamins, particularly B2 (riboflavin)

Vitamin B6 - Pyridoxine

RDI: 1.3–1.7 mg

DEFINITION

Vitamin B6 also known as Pyridoxine is a water soluble vitamin that performs a wide variety of functions in the body. An important one for those concerned with protein and bodybuilding.

FOODS I'D RECOMMEND

- Sesame seeds (100 g - 0.79 mg)
- Almond nuts (100 g - 0.14 mg)
- Sweet Potatoes (100 g - 0.2 mg)
- Teff (1 cup - 0.9 mg)
- Hemp seeds (100 g - 0.6 mg)
- Amaranth* (1 cup - 1.1 mg)

- Spinach (100 g - 0.2 mg)

- Pistachios (100 g - 1.7 mg)

- Bananas (100 g - 0.4 mg)

- Avocados (100 g - 0.3 mg)

*uncooked statistic

BENEFITS

- Red blood cell production

- Liver detoxification

- Brain and nervous system health

- Anti inflammatory

- Improved mood

DEFICIENCY SYMPTOMS

Some symptoms include:

- Scaling on the lipsSwollen tongue
- Confusion
- Weakened immune function
- Fatigue
- Pins and needles

RELATES TO

- Vitamin B12
- Folic acid.
- B3

Vitamin B9 - Folate

RDI: 0.4 mg

DEFINITION

Vitamin B9, also known as Folate, is important for brain health and it plays an important role in mental and emotional health.

FOODS I'D RECOMMEND

- Pecan nuts (100 g - 0.022 mg)
- Chickpeas (100 g - 0.172 mg)
- Lentils (100 g - 0.1 mg)
- Black eyed beans (100 g - 0.352 mg)
- Spinach (100 g - 0.194 mg)
- Asparagus (100 g - 0.052 mg)
- Okra (100 g - 0.272 mg)
- Sea moss (100 g - 0.182)
- Hemp seeds (20 g - 0.022 mg)

BENEFITS

- DNA synthesis and repair
- Cell division, and cell growth
- Creation of white and red blood cells
- May help prevent some cancers

DEFICIENCY SYMPTOMS

- Poor growth
- Tongue inflammation
- Gingivitis
- Loss of appetite
- Shortness of breath
- Diarrhea
- Irritability
- Forgetfulness
- Mental sluggishness

Vitamin B12 - Cobalamin

RDI: 0.0024 mg

DEFINITION

Unlike other B Vitamins, Vitamin B12 can be stored in the body for several years. No plant or animal can make vitamin B12. It's only microorganisms like fungi and bacteria can that do, hence why B12 is found in soil and, it is typically only animal foods that contain B12 due to their eating habits. There are some foods that are said to have B12 but it's worth noting that the percent of vitamin B12 your body can absorb from supplements is not very high.

Below are some of my go to sources but I also own a supplement.

FOODS I'D RECOMMEND

- Dulse Seaweed (100 g - 0.066 mg)
- Duckweed (100 g - 0.00212 mg)
- Sea moss **
- Oyster Mushrooms (1 cup - 0.2 µg)
- Bladderwrack **
- Chlorella (30 g - 14.5-73 µg)
- Nori Seaweed, dried from japan (30 g - 4.3 µg)
- Kelp (30 g - 1.2 µg)

**little to no information found of B12 levels

BENEFITS

- Physical and emotional energy
- Mental clarity
- Concentration and memory mood regulation
- Healthy nervous system

- Female reproductive health

- Pregnancy health

- Adrenal hormone production

- Proper circulation

- Cell formation

DEFICIENCY SYMPTOMS

- Weakness

- Tiredness or lightheartedness

- Heart palpitations

- Shortness of breath

- Pale skin

- A smooth tongue

- Constipation

- Diarrhoea

- Pins and needles

- Loss of appetite or gas

- Numbness

- Muscle weakness and problems walking

- Vision loss

- Depression
- Memory loss

EXTRA TIPS

If deficient, get tested and supplement. B12 is produced in the gut, which many believe is too far in your digestive process to get absorbed by the body. The best thing to do is ensure absorption is to look after your holistic health, and your gut! You can look after your gut by being mindful of how much food you eat that is high in sugar, gluten or is processed.. No matter what diet you choose, chances are you may need to pay close attention to this nutrient.

Vitamin C

RDI: 90 mg

DEFINITION

Vitamin C, also known as ascorbic acid and ascorbate, is an essential nutrient involved in the repair of tissue and the enzymatic production of certain neurotransmitters. It is required for the biosynthesis of collagen and L-carnitine, also, vitamin C is also involved in protein metabolism.

FOODS I'D RECOMMEND

- Orange
- Blackcurrants
- Orange juice
- Red and green Peppers
- Strawberries
- Broccoli

- Brussels

- Sprouts

- Lemons

BENEFITS

- Boosts Immune system

- Good mood

- Wound repair

- Cure lead toxicity

- Bone health

- Helps iron deficiency

- Helps manage high blood pressure

DEFICIENCY SYMPTOMS

- Bumpy skin

- Swollen joints

- Spoon shaped fingernails

Helps increase iron absorption

Vitamin D

RDI: 25–100 micrograms

DEFINITION

Vitamin D is required for the absorption of calcium, bone development, immune functioning, and alleviation of inflammation. Vitamin D can be broken down into two types, Vitamin D2 and D3.

D2 or ergocalciferol is synthesised by plants and is not produced by the human body. Whereas D3 or cholecalciferol is made in large quantities in the skin when sunlight strikes bare skin. It can also be ingested from animal sources.

FOODS I'D RECOMMEND

- Mushrooms* (100 g - 2300 micrograms)
- Sunlight

BENEFITS

- Maintains the health of bones and teeth
- Boost immune system, brain and nervous system
- Regulates insulin levels
- Supports lung function and cardiovascular health
- Bone and teeth health

DEFICIENCY SYMPTOMS

- Weakened immune system
- Seasonal depression
- Autoimmune disease
- Risks of cancer
- Weak bones
- Skin issues like eczema

RELATES TO

Vitamin D is necessary for the absorption of calcium and regulating the absorption of phosphorus. Also, Vitamin D is oil soluble, which means you need to eat fat to absorb it. If you do supplement, ensure it's fat soluble supplement, good supplements may have some fat, like coconut oil, in the pill.

Vitamin E

RDI: 15 mg

DEFINITION

Vitamin E is a fat soluble compound.

FOODS I'D RECOMMEND

- Almonds (28 g - 6.8 mg)
- Cashews (100 g - 0.9 mg)
- Sunflower seeds (28 g - 7.4 mg)
- Spinach (100 g - 2.3 mg)
- Hemp seeds (100 g - 15.4 mg)
- Quinoa (100 g - 8.7 mg)
- Kale (100 g - 1.54 mg)
- Hazelnuts (28 g - 4.3 mg)
- Broccoli (1 cup - 2.4 mg)

BENEFITS

- Reduces oxidative stress
- Beneficial for skin
- Anti ageing
- May reduce high blood pressure

DEFICIENCY SYMPTOMS

Vitamin E deficiency, which is rare and is usually due to an underlying problem with digesting dietary fat rather than from a diet low in vitamin E. Symptoms may inclue:

- Mild anemia
- infertility
- Fragile red blood cells
- Age spots
- Cataracts
- Decrease in sex drive
- Muscle, liver and brain function abnormalities

- Gastrointestinal diseases

- Hair loss

- Muscular weakness

- Slow tissue healing

- Leg cramps

Vitamin H - Biotin

RDI: 0.03mg

DEFINITION

Vitamin H, also known as Biotin or Vitamin B7 is a water-soluble B-complex vitamin that helps the body metabolise proteins and process glucose.

FOODS I'D RECOMMEND

- Legumes (100 g - 0.023 mg)
- Spinach (1/2 cup - 0.0003 mg)
- Almonds (1/2 cup - 0.003 mg)
- Sunflower seeds (1/2 cup - 0.0052 mg)
- Avocado (100 g - 0.0032 - 0.01 mg)
- Sweet potato (half cup - 0.0024 mg)
- Broccoli (half cup - 0.0004 mg)

- Cauliflower (100g - 0.017 mg)

- Bananas (half cup - 0.004 mg)

- Mushrooms (100g - 0.016 mg)

BENEFITS

- Strengthens hair

- Improves skin health

- Helps metabolism

- Aids in lowering cholesterol

- Helps regulate blood sugar

DEFICIENCY SYMPTOMS

- Biotin deficiencies are rare.

EXTRA TIPS

Cooking or heat can make biotin ineffective.

Less-processed foods may contain more active biotin.

Vitamin K

RDI: 0.12 mg for women and 0.38 mg for men

DEFINITION

Vitamin K is a group of compounds, including Vitamin K1 and vitamin K2.

FOODS I'D RECOMMEND

- Spinach (100 g - 0.541 mg)
- Asparagus (100 g - 0.081 mg)
- Strawberries (100 g - 0.0022 mg)
- Broccoli (½ cup - 0.11 mg)

BENEFITS

- Bone health
- Blood pressure

Minerals

[**min**-er-*uh* l, **min**-r*uh* l]

Minerals are found in the earth and hold on to their chemical structure. They play an important role in growth, bone health, fluid balance and several other processes.

Calcium

RDI: 1000 - 1200 mg

DEFINITION

Calcium is necessary for strong teeth and bones. Also it plays an important role in muscle contraction and secretion of certain hormones. Most of the calcium in the body is in our bones and teeth.

FOODS I'D RECOMMEND

- Watercress (100 g - 81 mg)
- Poppy seeds (1 tbsp - 126 mg)
- White beans (1 cup - 169 mg)
- Lentils (100 g - 19 mg)
- Kale (100 g - 150 mg)
- Okra (100 g - 82 mg)
- Hemp seeds (20 g - 14 mg)

- Broccoli (100 g - 47 mg)

- Almonds (100 g - 288 mg)

- Rhubarb** (100 g - 86 mg)

- Cashews (100 g - 37mg)

- Cacao (100 g - 128 mg)

- Oats (100 g - 631 mg)

**Green vegetables can be high in oxalates which can reduce calcium absorption, boiling can help reduce the oxalates.

BENEFITS

Your body needs calcium to:

- Build and maintain strong bones

- Heart health

- Optimal muscles contraction and nerves function

DEFICIENCY SYMPTOMS

- Numbness in fingers and toes

- Muscle cramps and aches
- Convulsions
- Lethargy
- Loss of appetite
- Abnormal heart rhythms
- Premenstrual cramps
- Vitamin D deficiency
- Hypertension and arthritis.

RELATES TO

Vitamin D, C, E, K, magnesium, and boron help the body absorb calcium.

Copper

RDI: 1 - 1.7 mg

DEFINITION

Copper is required by the body for bone and connective tissue production..

FOODS I'D RECOMMEND

- Lentils (100 g - 0.35 mg)
- Brazil nuts (28 g - 0.5 mg)
- Almonds (100 g - 1.03 mg)
- Chickpeas (100 g - 0.85 mg)
- Cashews Nuts (100 g - 2.19 mg)
- Teff (1 cup - 17.8 mg)
- Mushrooms (100 g - 0.14 mg)
- Quinoa (100 g - 0.19 mg)
- Black eyed beans (100 g - 0.21 mg)
- Cacao powder (100 g - 3.79 mg)

- Watermelon seeds (100 g - 0.69 mg)
- Flax seeds (100 g - 1.22 mg)
- Avocado (1 whole - 0.3 mg)

BENEFITS

- Supports neurodevelopment and growth
- Boosts immune system benefits
- Helps form red blood cells
- Prevent cardiovascular diseases
- Contributes to iron absorption
- Better energy
- Beneficial for skin health

DEFICIENCY SYMPTOMS

- Joint pain
- Fatigue
- Premature grey hair
- Memory and concentration issues

- Sensitivity to cold

- Lowered immunity

- Anemia

- Hypertension

- Inflammation

RELATES TO

Iron absorption

Iron

RDI: 8 mg

DEFINITION

Iron is an important nutrient for optimal health, it's essential to help carry oxygen within the body. The two forms of iron are heme and nonheme iron. Heme iron is mainly found in animals whilst plants provide only nonheme form of iron.

FOODS I'D RECOMMEND

- Spinach (1 cup - 0.81 mg)
- Broccoli (1 cup - 0.66 mg)
- Lentils (100 g - 3.3 mg)
- Thyme (1 teaspoon - 1.2 mg)
- Navy beans (100 g - 2.4 mg)
- Apricots (100 g - 0.36

- Teff (1 cup - 14.7 mg)

- Cashews (100 g - 6 mg)

- Hemp seeds (100 g - 3.9 mg)

- Chia seeds (100 g - 7.72 mg)

- Amaranth (1 cup - 14.7 mg)

- Hemp seeds (20 g - 1.59 mg)

- Kale (100 g - 0.94 mg)

- Basil (100 g - 3.2 mg)

- Nettle powder (100 g - 277 mg)

- Cacao powder(100 g - 13.86 mg)

- Sea moss (100 g - 8.9 mg)

- Avocado (1 whole - 0.9 mg)

- Figs (100 g - 0.37 mg)

BENEFITS

- Better concentration & focus

- Regulation of body temperature

- Energy

- Hair health

- Hemoglobin formation

- Oxygen carrier
- Muscle health
- Brain health

DEFICIENCY SYMPTOMS

- Anemia
- Fatigue
- Heart palpitations
- Pale skin
- Shortness of breath
- Poor hair health
- Cravings
- Pins and needles
- Tongue swelling or soreness
- Cold hands and feet
- Brittle nails
- Headaches
- Poor concentration
- Weakened immune system
- Leaky gut or IBS

RELATES TO

Choose foods containing vitamin C to enhance iron absorption.

Magnesium

RDI: 310–420 mg

DEFINITION

Magnesium is needed for more than 300 biochemical reactions in the body including nerve signaling, the building of healthy bones, and normal muscle contraction. Magnesium deficiency is often associated with low blood levels of calcium and potassium.

FOODS I'D RECOMMEND

- Cashews (100 g - 260 mg)
- Spinach (100 g - 76 mg)
- Avocado (100 g - 29 mg)
- Brazil nuts (28 g - 106 mg)
- Quinoa (100 g - 64 mg)
- Watermelon seeds (1 cup - 556 mg)
- Kale (100 g - 47 mg)

- Lentils (100 g - 36 mg)

- Chickpeas (100 g - 48 mg)

- Teff (1 cup - 455 mg)

- Amaranth (1 cup - 479 mg)

- Bananas (100 g- 27 mg)

- Banana chips (100 g - 76 mg)

- Cacao or dark chocolate (100 g - 228 mg)

- Figs (100 g - 17 mg)

- Pumpkin seeds (28 g - 150 mg)

- Sea moss (100 g - 144 mg)

BENEFITS

- Energy

- Protein formation

- Muscle movement

- Increased sports performance

- Good brain function

- Good mood

- Anti-inflammatory

- Blood pressure benefits

- May prevent headaches
- Improves PMS symptoms

DEFICIENCY SYMPTOMS

- Muscle twitches
- Eye twitching
- Irregular heartbeat
- Lack of motivation
- Poor appetite

RELATES TO

Calcium and Vitamin D.

Manganese

RDI: 2.5 to 3 mg

DEFINITION

Manganese is required by the body to aid in nutrient absorption along with many other processes such as enzyme functions, wound healing, and bone development.

FOODS I'D RECOMMEND

- Hazelnuts (100 g - 6.18 mg)
- Cashews (100 g - 1.66 mg)
- Almonds (100 g - 2.23 mg)
- Avocado (1 whole - 0.3 mg)
- Watermelon seeds (1 cup - 1.7 mg)
- Cacao (100 g - 3.84 mg)
- Teff (1 cup - 17.8 mg)
- Amaranth* (1 cup - 6.4 mg)

- Ground Cloves (100 g - 60.127 mg)

- Ground Ginger (100 g - 33.3 mg)

- Chickpeas (100 g - 1.03 mg)

- Oats (100 g - 2.2 mg)

*uncooked statistic

BENEFITS

- Strengthens weak bones

- Antioxidant

- Alleviates PMS symptoms

- Fights anemia

- Reduces inflammation

- Improves alopecia

- Improve bone health

- Blood sugar regulation

DEFICIENCY SYMPTOMS

Manganese deficiency is rare but symptoms can be seen expressed in:

- Poor bone health
- Joint pain
- Fertility problems.
- High blood pressure
- Poor eyesight
- Hearing trouble
- Memory loss

Phosphorus

RDI: 700 mg

DEFINITION

Phosphorus is an essential nutrient needed for cell functioning along with many other body processes.

FOODS I'D RECOMMEND

- Pumpkin seeds ** (100 g - 1233 mg)
- Dulse seaweed (100 g - 414 mg)
- Kelp seaweed (100 g - 428 mg)
- Oats (1 cup - 816 mg)
- Watermelon seeds (1 cup - 815 mg)
- Hemp seeds (20 g - 330 mg)
- Teff (1 cup - 828 mg)
- Chia seeds (100 g - 946 mg)
- Cashew nuts ** (1/2 cup - 280 mg)

- Brazil nuts (1/2 cup - 462 mg)

- Lentils** (1 cup - 250 mg)

- Chickpeas (1 cup - 274 mg)

**up to 80% of the phosphorus found in nuts & seeds is in a stored form called phytic acid, or phytate, which humans cannot digest. To reduce this percentage soak them until they sprout and cook with them.

BENEFITS

- Healthy bone formation
- Improved digestion
- Better bowel movements
- Protein formation
- Hormonal balance
- Healthy hair
- DNA health

DEFICIENCY SYMPTOMS

- Decreased appetite

- Anemia

- Muscle pain

- Numbness

- Weakened immune system

- Fatigue

- Joint stiffness

- Anxiety

RELATES TO

Calcium or magnesium.

Iodine

RDI: 0.2 mcg

DEFINITION

Iodine is an important mineral found in some foods. The body needs iodine to make thyroid hormones. Thyroid hormones control the body's metabolism and are important in weight management.

FOODS I'D RECOMMEND

- Dulse seaweed (7 g - 1.169 mg)
- Sea moss (100 g - 0.8 mg)
- Lugols supplement
- Nori seaweed (100 g - 1.6 mg)
- Kelp (7 g - 3.17 mg)
- Lima beans** (1 cup - 0.016 mg)

**Cooked

BENEFITS

- Promotes thyroid health
- Weight management
- Improves cognitive function
- Improves immune system

DEFICIENCY SYMPTOMS

- Enlarged thyroid gland (goitre)
- Tiredness
- Weight-gain
- Increased susceptibility to infections
- Depression
- Feeling cold at extremities
- Dry and cracked skin

EXTRA INFORMATION

Foods that contain goitrogens interfere with iodine absorption. Foods high in goitrogens include soy, cassava and cabbage

Potassium

RDI: 3500–4700 mg

DEFINITION

Potassium is an important electrolyte, it's needed to help muscles contract and it helps the heart beat properly.

FOODS I'D RECOMMEND

- Bananas (1 large - 487 mg)
- Lentils (1 cup - 730.6 mg)
- Watermelon (1 cup - 170 mg)
- Spinach (1 cup - 540 mg)
- Hemp seeds (20 g - 240 mg)
- Sweet Potatoes (100 g - 337 mg)
- Avocado (100 g - 485 mg)
- Mushrooms (100 g - 318 mg)

- Kelp seaweed (100 g - 11200 mg)

- Dulse (100 g - 7814 mg)

- Figs (100 g - 242 mg)

- White beans (1 cup - 829 mg)

BENEFITS

- Blood pressure benefits

- Heart and kidney benefits

- Reduces anxiety and stress

- Enhances muscle strength

- Regulates metabolism

- Nervous system benefits

DEFICIENCY SYMPTOMS

- Fatigue

- Muscle weakness

- Abnormal heartbeat

- Heart palpitations

- Anemia

- Severe headaches

- High blood pressure

- Pain in their intestines

- Muscle cramps and spasms

- Digestive problems

- Pins and needles

RELATES TO

Calcium

Selenium

RDI: 0.055 - 0.07 mg

DEFINITION

Selenium is an essential trace mineral important for cognitive function, a healthy immune system and fertility for both men and women.

FOODS I'D RECOMMEND

- Brazil nuts (28 g - 0.542 mg)
- Chia seeds ** (100 g - 0.0552 mg)
- Mushrooms (100 g - 0.012 mg)
- Cashew nuts (28 g - 0.003 mg)
- Lentils (1 cup - 0.002 mg)
- Oats (1 cup - 0.013 mg)

**Soak to increase absorption

BENEFITS

- Essential for testosterone
- Boosts immune system
- Reproductive health
- Antioxidant
- Thyroid health
- Brain health

DEFICIENCY SYMPTOMS

- Pain in the muscles and joints
- White spots on nails
- Hair loss
- Mental fog
- Muscle weakness
- Weakened immune system
- Infertility

Zinc

RDI: 8 - 11 mg

DEFINITION

Zinc plays a role in immune system processes, protein synthesis, wound healing and cell division.

FOODS I'D RECOMMEND

- Spinach (100 g - 0.76 mg)
- Kidney beans (1/2 cup - 0.9 mg)
- Flax (100 g - 4.34 mg)
- Watermelon Seeds (1 cup - 11.1 mg)
- Chickpeas (100 g - 3.43 mg)
- Cashews (28 g - 1.6 mg)
- Mushrooms (1 cup - 1.4 mg)
- Pumpkin seeds (1/4 cup - 2.52 mg)
- Hemp seeds (20 g - 1.98 zinc)

- Kelp (100 g - 2.85 mg)

- Dulse (100 g - 2.85 mg)

- Cacao (100 g - 6.1 mg)

BENEFITS

- Immune system

- Antioxidant

- Hormonal balance

- Digestion & nutrient absorption

- Liver health

- Muscle Growth and Repair

- Brain health

- Faster wound healing

DEFICIENCY SYMPTOMS

- Changes in appetite

- Food cravings for salty or sweet foods

- Changes in ability to taste and smell

- Weight gain or loss

- Hair loss

- Digestive problems

- Fatigue

- Infertility

- Hormonal problems

- Low immunity

- Poor concentration and memory

RELATES TO

Magnesium helps the body regulate zinc levels. Additionally, zinc enables the body to absorb magnesium more efficiently

Protein

[**proh**-teen, -tee-in]

Protein is crucial for growth and repair. Protein is made up of 22 amino acids, when protein is broken down, these amino acids are left. Amino acids are grouped in two main classes: essential and nonessential.

There are 9 essential amino acids. These are amino acids that cannot be made by the body and must be obtained from the diet. On the other hand, there are 13 non-essential amino acids. These can be made by the body from essential amino acids and other cofactors. We will discuss essential amino acids in following chapters.

The cofactors include enzymes, vitamins, minerals and other amino acids. If these are missing, the body cannot produce the 'non-essential' amino acid. That's another reason why you should ensure you're getting all your nutrient needs, it's essential for protein.

The subsequent chapters should help with your essential protein sources.

Histidine

RDI: 18 mg per gram of protein

DEFINITION

Histidine is an essential amino acid required for growth and tissue repair, blood cell production, and creation of histamine.

FOODS I'D RECOMMEND

- Navy beans (1 cup - 542 mg)
- Pumpkin seeds (100 g - 770 mg)
- Hemp seeds (4.8 mg per gram)
- Peanut butter (2 tbsp - 178 mg)
- Watermelon seeds (100 g - 775 mg)
- Sunflower seeds powder (100 g - 1333 mg)
- Peanuts (100 g - 480 mg)
- Sesame seeds (100 g - 536 mg)
- Almonds (100 g - 615 mg)

- Chia seeds (100 g - 526 mg)

- Pistachio (100 g - 507 mg)

- Chickpeas (100 g - 0.24 g)

- Flax (100 g - 472 mg)

- Lentils (1 cup - 503 mg)

- Red kidney beans (1 cup - 467 mg)

- Cashew nuts (100 g - 0.46 g)

- Quinoa (3.2 g per 100g protein)

- Teff (100 g - 0.3 mg)

BENEFITS

- Protect tissues from damage

- Improved sex drive

- Reduction in allergies

- Regulates blood ph

- Improves nerve cells

- Help create hormones

- Tissue repair

- Brain health

- **Help break down trace elements like copper and iron

DEFICIENCY SYMPTOMS

- Eczema
- Anemia
- Pneumonia
- Ulcers

Cysteine

RDI: 25 mg per gram of protein

DEFINITION

Cysteine is an amino acid which can generally be manufactured by the body. Cysteine is synthesised from methionine.

FOODS I'D RECOMMEND

- Chia seeds
- Quinoa (4.8 g per 100 g protein)
- Hemp seeds (100 g - 0.672 g)
- Brazil nuts
- Chickpeas (100 g - 0.12 g)
- Lentils
- Teff (100 g - 0.24 mg)

BENEFITS

- Kidney health
- Brain health
- Helps create antioxidants
- Liver health
- Improve fertility in men and women
- May be antiinflammatory
- Immune system boost

DEFICIENCY SYMPTOMS

- Lack of motivation
- Grey hair
- Sluggish
- Liver damage
- Muscle loss
- Skin lesions
- Weakness
- Fat loss
- Slowed growth in children

Isoleucine

RDI: 25 mg per gram of protein

DEFINITION

Isoleucine is a branched-chain amino acid (BCAA). There are three branched-chain amino acids in the body, these are isoleucine, valine, and leucine. BCAAs have been shown to build muscle, decrease muscle fatigue and alleviate muscle soreness. Isoleucine is mainly concentrated in the muscle tissues.

FOODS I'D RECOMMEND

- Lentils (100 g - 390 mg)
- Kamut (100 g - 220 mg)
- Pumpkin seeds (100 g - 1265 mg)
- Hemp seeds* (28 g - 365 mg)
- Pistachio (28 g - 272 mg)
- Cashew butter (28 g - 238 mg)

- Cashew (28 g - 224 mg)

- Black eyed beans (1 cup - 527 mg)

- Navy beans (1 cup - 933 mg)

- Lentils (1 cup - 733 mg)

- Kidney beans (1 cup - 726 mg)

- Mung beans (1 cup - 693 mg)

- Spirulina (100 g - 3.21 mg)

- Chickpeas (1 cup - 623 mg)

- Spinach (100 g - 0.14 mg)

- Teff (100 g - 0.5 g)

- Quinoa (4.4 g per 100 g protein)

- Almonds (28 g - 212 mg)

*Hemp powder is more concentrated (50% protein)

BENEFITS

- Aid in muscle recovery

- Helps endurance

- Aids in building muscle

- Boost energy

- Lowers glucose

DEFICIENCY SYMPTOMS

- Dizziness
- Fatigue
- Headaches
- Confusion
- Irritability
- Depression

Leucine

RDI: 55 mg per gram of protein

DEFINITION

Leucine is another branched-chain amino acid (BCAA). It is used in the liver, fat tissue, and muscle tissue and it is unique in its ability to stimulate skeletal muscle protein synthesis. In fact, leucine at a very high dose can stimulate muscle protein synthesis.

FOODS I'D RECOMMEND

- Kamut (100 g - 0.43 g)
- Cashew nuts (100 g - 1.47 g)
- Mung Beans (100 g - 0.54 g)
- Chickpeas (100 g - 0.63 g)
- Sweet Potatoes (100 g - 0.12 g)
- Flax (100 g - 1.24 g)
- Teff (100 g - 1.07 g)
- Hemp seeds (100 g - 2.163 mg)

- Cashews Nuts (100 g - 1.47 g)

- Macadamia nuts (100 g - 0.6 g)

- Pistachio (100 g - 1.6 g)

- Quinoa (6.6 g per 100 g protein)

- Chia seeds (100 g - 1.37 g)

BENEFITS

- Leucine stimulates protein Synthesis

- Increased muscle growth

- Decreased muscle soreness (DOMS)

- Reduces exercise fatigue

- Beneficial for liver health

- Maximise muscle anabolism after exercise

- Aids fat loss

- Helps with cholesterol control

DEFICIENCY SYMPTOMS

- Decreased appetite
- Sluggish
- Headaches
- Hair loss
- Dizziness
- Fatigue
- Depression
- Confusion
- Irritability.

Lysine

RDI: 51 mg per gram of protein

DEFINITION

Lysine is involved in collagen creation and the absorption of calcium.

FOODS I'D RECOMMEND

- Chia seeds (100 g - 0.970 g)
- Chickpeas (100 g - 0.59 g)
- Quinoa (6.1 g per 100 g protein)
- Cashew nuts (100 g - 0.93 g)
- Hemp seeds (100 g - 1.273 mg)
- Black eyed beans (100 g - 0.21 g)
- Lentils (100 g - 0.630 g)
- Kamut (100 g - 0.16 g)
- Teff (100 g - 0.38 g)
- Amaranth

- Pistachio (100 g - 1.2 g)

BENEFITS

- Reduce anxiety
- Improve calcium absorption
- Boost immune system, skin
- Promote bone health
- Promote normal growth
- Helps convert fatty acids to energy
- Promotes wound healing
- Improved muscle strength and performance
- Aids weight loss

DEFICIENCY SYMPTOMS

- Fatigue
- Poor concentration
- Hair Loss
- Stunted growth

- Bloodshot eyes

- Anorexia

RELATES TO

Absorption of calcium.

Methionine

RDI: 25 mg per gram of protein

DEFINITION

Methionine is an essential amino acid. It may help prevent hair loss

FOODS I'D RECOMMEND

- Brazil nuts (100 g - 1.124 mg)
- Almonds (100 g - 0.16 g)
- Quinoa (4.8 g per 100 g protein)
- Cashew nuts (100 g - 0.36 g)
- Hemp seeds (100 g - 0.933 mg)
- Chia seeds (100 g - 0.588 g)
- Teff (100 g - 0.43 g)
- Spelt (100 g - 0.26)
- Chickpeas (100 g - 0.12 g)
- White beans (1 cup - 261 mg)

- Red kidney beans (1 cup - 254 mg)

BENEFITS

- Synthesis of L-cysteine
- Antioxidant
- Liver health
- Improved wound healing
- Used to produce important molecules
- Production of DNA
- Metabolism of nutrients

DEFICIENCY SYMPTOMS

- Apathy
- Grey hair
- Muscle loss
- Fat loss
- Weakness

RELATES TO

Supports the absorption of selenium and zinc.

EXTRA TIPS

Some experts believe it's best to keep consumption of Methionine low. This may be to do with some studies showing that some cancer cells are dependent on dietary methionine to grow. Additionally, several studies in animals show that reducing methionine can increase lifespan and improve health.

Phenylalanine

RDI: 47 mg per gram of protein

DEFINITION

Phenylalanine is an essential amino acid involved in many body processes. Some processes include creating DNA, dopamine and the skin pigment melanin. The body can also use Phenylalanine to make the amino acid tyrosine.

FOODS I'D RECOMMEND

- Cashew nuts (100 g - 0.93 g)
- Pistachio (100 g - 1.11 g)
- Chia seeds (100 g - 1.016 g)
- Almonds (100 g - 1.13 g)
- Hemp seeds (100 g - 1.447 mg)
- Lentils (100 g - 0.43 mg)
- Teff (100 g - 0.7 g)

- Kamut (100 g - 0.3 g)

- Spelt (100 g - 0.74 g)

- Quinoa (7.3 g per 100 g protein)

- Chickpeas (100 g - 0.48 g)

- Amaranth (100 g - 0.54 g)

- Mung Beans (100 g - 0.01 g)

BENEFITS

- Promotes alertness

- Aids appetite control

- Improves memory

- Improves mood

- Anti Inflammatory

- Skin benefits

DEFICIENCY SYMPTOMS

- Confusion

- Lack of energy

- Reduced alertness

- Reduced Memory
- Lack of appetite.

Threonine

RDI: 27 mg per gram of protein

DEFINITION

Threonine supports cardiovascular, liver, central nervous, and immune system functions.

FOODS I'D RECOMMEND

- Peanuts (100 g - 0.61 g)
- White beans (1 cup - 735 mg)
- Cashew nuts (100 g - 0.69 g)
- Chia seeds (100 g - 0.709 g)
- Hemp seeds (100 g - 1.269 mg)
- Chickpeas (100 g - 0.33 g)
- Teff (100 g - 0.51 g)
- Quinoa (3.8 g per 100 g protein)

BENEFITS

- Supports the immune system
- Supports liver function
- Supports nervous system
- Digestive system health

DEFICIENCY SYMPTOMS

- Emotional agitation
- Digestion difficulties

RELATES TO

Needed to create glycine and serine.

Tryptophan

RDI: 7 mg per gram of protein

DEFINITION

Tryptophan is an essential amino acid needed for general growth and development within the body. Tryptophan also helps create niacin. Niacin is essential in creating serotonin which helps control your mood and sleep.

FOODS I'D RECOMMEND

- Chia seeds (100 g - 0.463 g)
- Chickpeas (100 g - 0.09 g)
- Sesame seeds (100 g - 0.37 g)
- Sunflower (100 g - 0.27 g)
- Flax seeds (100 g - 0.23 g)
- Hemp seeds (100 g - 0.369 mg)
- Teff (100 g - 0.14 g)

- Quinoa (1.1 g per 100 g protein)

- Pistachio (100 g - 0.27 g)

- Cashew nuts (100 g - 0.29 g)

- Lentils (100 g - 0.22 g)

BENEFITS

- Boost sleep quality

- Better mood

- Beneficial for brain health

- Aids appetite control

- Potential in fighting depression & anxiety

- Boosts memory

DEFICIENCY SYMPTOMS

- Insomnia

- Cravings of carbohydrates

- Depression

- Inability to concentrate

- Irritability

Valine

RDI: 32 mg per gram of protein

DEFINITION

Valine is one of the three branched-chain amino acids, which means it can provide muscles with energy. The amino acid valine is an essential amino acid that is used in the biosynthesis of proteins.

FOODS I'D RECOMMEND

- Lentils (100 g - 0.62)
- Broccoli (100 g - 0.13 g)
- Kidney beans (100 g - 1.23 g)
- Chickpeas (100 g - 0.37 g)
- Cashew nuts (100 g - 1.09 g)
- Almonds (100 g - 0.94 g)
- Mushrooms (100 g - 0.14 g)

- Teff (100 g - 0.69 g)

- Hemp seeds (100 g - 1.777 mg)

- Quinoa (4.5 g per 100 g protein)

BENEFITS

- Muscle metabolism

- Muscle repair

- Calm mood

- Improve muscle coordination

- Promote normal growth, repair tissues

- Regulate blood sugar

- Aid central nervous system stimulation

- Needed for proper mental functioning.

Fats

[fats]

The body needs fat for energy and many of the body's processes but where do you get good fats on a vegan diet?

Firstly it's good to understand the types of fats.

There are monounsaturated fats (MUFA), polyunsaturated fats (PUFA), which are widely known as good fats. There are also trans fats and saturated fats which should be eaten in more limited quantities.

The important fats to be aware of are the Omegas. These are Omega 3, 7 and 9. The Omega-3 is the most useful. Omega 3 fatty acids are a type of PUFA and are especially beneficial to your health. There are different types of omega 3s, EPA and DHA, both of which can be gotten from food.

The following chapters will cover ALA and Omega 3. This is because the body, although less potent, converts a type of fat called ALA into EPA and DHA.

Omega 3

RDI: 250–500 mg

DEFINITION

Omega-3 fatty acids are very important fats for optimal health. The foods below are either DHA or ALA. Omega 3 supports heart, brain and eye health at all stages of life.

FOODS I'D RECOMMEND

- Chia seeds* 28 g - 5.055 g
- Nori **
- Wakame (1 cup - 18.8 mg)
- Dulse seaweed **
- Perilla Oil (14 g - 9000 mg)
- Brussels sprouts (1/2 cup - 135 g)
- Walnuts (1 tbsp - 3.346 g)
- Sea moss (100 g - 47 mg)

- Flax seeds* (1 tbsp - 6.703 g)

- Oats (100 g - 17552 mg)

- Hemp seeds (3 tbsp - 2.605 g)

**Data not found

* Can also get oils too

BENEFITS

- Boosts immune system

- Anti-inflammatory

- Improved eye health

- Boosts brain health

- Reduce blood pressure

- Bone and joint health

DEFICIENCY SYMPTOMS

- Dry skin and hair and soft or brittle nails

- Rough patches of skin

- Small bumps

- Eczema
- Attention Deficit
- Inability to concentrate
- Anxiety
- Mood swings
- Fatigue
- Poor sleep quality
- Joint pain.

ALA

RDI: 1.6 grams for men and 1.1 grams for women

DEFINITION

Our bodies can't make ALA (alpha-linolenic acid) so we must get it from food. You can easily meet their ALA needs by consuming a little ground chia or ground flax seeds every day. I prefer chia to flax for its other benefits. Be mindful that although ALA is a precursor to EPA and DHA, the conversion percentage can be quite low.

FOODS I'D RECOMMEND

- Macadamia nuts
- Hemp seeds oil
- Chia seeds
- Flax seeds

- Walnuts
- Cashews Nuts
- Avocado

Help me help you

Thank you so much for purchasing this guide, I hope it has been useful for you. I want you to help me spread the message. Please make sure you leave reviews, share this guide with friends and shout from the rooftops to let the world know.

Being armed with knowledge and a step by step guide to apply the knowledge brings power and confidence to those embarking on new lifestyle changes.

I'm looking forward to seeing all the recipes you create with these foods. Be sure to tag me on instagram @dungubook.

Remember this is not an exhaustive list of foods, there are thousands of potential foods. If you come across some interesting foods or you just wish to share your thoughts with me, drop me a note at paul@dungubook.com. Until next time. Stay healthy.

Health is wealth,

Paul Otote